BIODYNAMICS OF OSTEOPATHY

Phase Three

Second Edition

James Jealous D.O.

For more information about Dr. Jealous please visit:
https://BiodynamicsOfOsteopathy.com

BIODYNAMICS OF OSTEOPATHY   Phase Three

Hardback ISBN: 979-8-2955-3921-3

Second Edition 2025

James Jealous D.O. (1943–2021) practiced as an osteopathic physician, teacher and writer for many years. His life's work was to found and develop the specific methodology of Biodynamics of Osteopathy, following the lineage of Dr. A.T. Still and Dr. W.G. Sutherland.

This is one of a series of Biodynamics of Osteopathy books. They grew organically from sets of handouts written by Dr. Jealous and given to students during courses taught by him and his teachers. After many years he collected the handouts together and created individual course manuals, which he added to and rewrote many times. After several more years they evolved further into books.

TABLE OF CONTENTS

OSTEOPATHY IS SERVICE viii
BE STILL AND KNOW 1
REVIEW OF PHASES ONE AND TWO 3
AUTOMATIC SHIFTING OVERVIEW 7
AUTOMATIC SHIFTING REVIEW 9
PHASE THREE OVERVIEW 12
THE POTENCY 14
THE SOFT POTENCY AND THE FLUID BODY 18
RESUSCITATION: EV4, SOFT POTENCY 20
MEDITATION: THE SEA AROUND US AND THROUGH US 21
THE MENINGES AND THE LONG-TIDE 22
THE MENINGEAL SACS 27
THE DURA MATER 29
TREATMENT 30
LANGUAGE, PHASE THREE 31
SEGMENTATION OF THE DURA MATER 34
THE SEGMENTATION OF THE DURA 36
THE ANTERIOR DURAL GIRDLE 37
THE BIRD AND THE IMMUNE RESPONSE 38
THE NEUROBIOLOGICAL BASIS OF FEVER 43
THE STORY WITHIN 44
CHILDREN'S OBSERVATIONS 46
FATHER DURA 48
LONG-TIDE REFERENCES BY ROLLIN BECKER, D.O. 49
OSTEOPATHY – TAKING ITS RIGHTFUL PLACE 50

OSTEOPATHIC MAGAZINE, 1925 52
THE PAUSE AND THE LANGUAGE OF SILENCE 54
BIODYNAMICS OF OSTEOPATHY BOOK SERIES 57
ABOUT THE AUTHOR 63

OSTEOPATHY IS SERVICE

We use our hands . . .

To treat the Whole patient

To listen to the indwelling movements of Life

To treat all levels of illness

To assist in building the patient's functional reserve

To support homeostasis and trophicity by balancing the activity of the autonomic nervous system

To explore "laws not framed by human hands" (Dr. Still and Dr. Sutherland)

To cooperate and communicate with the Laws of Nature (Dr. Wales)

"To find the Health" (Dr. Still)

To get to the treatment plan

To get to the diagnosis

To help establish a point of Rest or Neutral around which the Whole can come to balance

To find Cause

We believe ...

We have an innate capacity to heal

The patient functions as a whole

The autonomic nervous system plays a major role in disease and healing

Structure and function are one form of activity

The Divine is indwelling

Life moves beyond death

There is a Constant Movement toward Normal

We are here to Serve Humanity

Normal is ...

"A sense of peace and harmony" (Dr. Sutherland)

Ease of motion, without tension

A capacity for Neutral

A sense of Wholeness to Life

The capacity for adaptation, change without compensation.

"Skill is proportionate to one's understanding of normal" (Dr. Still)

This Manual Is Dedicated To Rollin Becker, D.O.

Master Osteopath

Devoted Student Of Will Sutherland

Third-Generation Osteopath

Visionary Of The Long-Tide

Teacher Of Stillness

Of Love As The Vehicle Of Speech

Of Ease

Of Listening To A "Still Small Voice"

Of Being Centered By The Tide

Of Losing One's Ego

Of Neutral As The Beginning

May He Repose In Love Eternal

BE STILL AND KNOW

Recommended reading: *Be Still and Know.* Rollin E. Becker D.O. presented this talk in Philadelphia, Pennsylvania, on September 22, 1965. It is a dedication to William Garner Sutherland. Here is a brief quote from his presentation:

> Dr. Sutherland told us, 'I have often said that we lost something in Osteopathy that Dr. Still tried to get across, and that was the Spiritual ...'
> The Osteopathic concept concerns a living system and includes the cranial concept.
> We can sense something else not ordinarily mentioned in the anatomical-physiological texts of today. This is an overall tidal movement of the whole body, ...
> ... a physician should develop an objective awareness. ... He must be able to evaluate and determine diagnostic and prognostic insight ...
> ... the physician should have a subjective awareness of the potential for using the healing principles discussed herein.
> Be Still and Know" ... "You are getting back to Cause" ... "The Breath of Life is the fundamental principle in the science of Osteopathy.
> I would like to close with a quotation that is in a letter he sent me many years ago. ... 'Closer to me than breathing is the Creator of the cranial mechanism.... Closer to the patient is the Creator of his or her cranial mechanism ... My thinking-feeling-seeing-knowing fingers are guided Intelligently by the

Master Mechanic... It matters not what interpretation one may apply, providing one's mental trolley is on the wire.'

REVIEW OF PHASES ONE AND TWO

Phase One

Phase One began with the noticing of our mental and manual attitudes toward lesions. When we think of Osteopathy from the perspective of the Health and the ease in the patient, and not from the lesion and the inertia, the outcome and clarity of treatment is remarkable. This perspective is unique to our profession and yields great clinical success when appreciated.

We observed that seeing the parts is not the summit of our skills, but rather gaining a sense of Normality through Wholeness; that is our goal.

The role of Neutral as an expression of the Whole was paramount, and the history of it was briefly reviewed.

Motion Present was introduced as a means of engaging a therapeutic process without Motion Testing for Permitted Motion ... not to be more subtle or elite, but rather because the clinical outcomes improve in proportion to the synchronization of the operator with the indwelling motion, connected to the Health and the activities of respiration ... we called this The Thread ... a thread that connects the Lesion Field to the Health.

We reviewed the heroic effort of Sutherland to find and describe involuntary motion of the central nervous system (CNS). It moves in relationship to the third ventricle (Lamina Terminalis) ... we discovered that Sutherland was a visionary in this regard. Embryological research has proven his descriptions to be precise and beyond his time … even today his insights are just coming into view for those whose science explores the motion of growth and development.

Sutherland saw more with his hands than the microscope could or does see in Living Organisms. We discussed metabolic motion as the essential basis for cranial motion … This motion is the breathing of Primary Respiration in the tissues, fluids, and potencies of the whole … The Breath of Life catalyzes this motion by directing its own will and power into the creation of a rhythmic shape of movement … we call this inhalation and exhalation … a river of transmutation that heals, unfolds, and reorients our lives. Seen or unseen, The Tide transmutes inertia, creating motion present which has an internal disengagement, indwelling augmentation, synchronization, and a spatial orientation to the Health.

We Discussed the Zones.

We worked with balanced fluid tension (BFT), the treatment of Lesion Fields in the infant cranium, by addressing the Fluid Motion Present instead of the Tissue Motion Present. This leads to an ease in treatment that unveils a systemic response, Wholeness.

Rebalancing Was Stressed.

We also felt the Health in ourselves, as a daily meditation, letting the Health express itself.

Phase Two

Phase two centered upon the Fluid Body, a term we have created to support an understanding of the embryonic forces, Primary Respiration, and the activities we feel as we treat.

We discussed rates: the history and meaning behind a Polyrhythmic system.

"The Fluids can Lesion" is a landmark discovery by Sutherland. When Fluid Lesions, it feels like tissue and becomes Zone A.

The essential skill of sensing Zone A and Zone B as separate "bodies" was highlighted. We explored the Axial Fluctuations as described by W.G.S.

Repair of the Fluid Body is essential to healing, growth, and development.

We studied the relationship of Zone B to the Sea Around Us, noting that the Central Stillness of the Zones is a doorway.

Phase Two is *only* about the Laws appreciated at a two-to-three-cycles-per-minute rate in the patient.

We worked with Motion Present in the "tide" of the Fluid in the Fluid (potency, reciprocal tension potency, or direct and indirect current). We noted the direction of ease.

We discussed levels of Stillness.

We studied Automatic Shifting as a diagnostic and therapeutic tool.

Get the Fluids going first!

We saw the benefit of Dr. Becker's words: "Do not begin the treatment until the will of the patient surrenders to the Will of Primary Respiration." From his advice we found that "getting a Neutral is paramount to the workings of the Fluid Body and patient recovery as a Whole person, not just symptomatic relief."

Waiting becomes patience.

Neutral … Transmutation … Health!

"Skill Is Proportionate to Your Understanding of Normal."
Dr. Still

AUTOMATIC SHIFTING OVERVIEW

There are many forms of Automatic Shifting, each one unique to the level of the Potency that generates that particular process.

In Phase One we observed the diagnostics and therapeutics of Automatic Shifting at two to three cycles per minute in the Fluid Body.

These events are effects of Primary Respiration and its intended therapeutic force. We are watching the effect of a greater Mind at work.

As we continue our journey to find the Cause of Primary Respiration and our own Health, we must pass from seeing effects to searching for the therapeutic forces that generate these effects.

We are asking, "Where is the Fulcrum for this Landscape of Natural Laws?" … where is the origin or cause behind this Automatic Shifting and its precision that knows the patient better than we do?

The task is to "turn the page in the story of the moment and read on."

Automatic Shifting is inside Zone B … The therapeutic forces are coming from Zone D or beyond … sensing inside and outside as you work will "turn the page in the next chapter of the Story." … Where is the power that generates this caring that is so geometrical and circumstantial? It is as if one is known.

The precursor to Automatic Shifting is a Neutral Fluid Body. The Stillpoint that ends the treatment fills a Space greater than Zone B.

Often the little lesions are treated first … to gather the energy to transmute the larger lesions …

The treatment continues to maturate for at least seventy-two hours.

According to Alan Becker, it takes thirty-six and a half hours for the lesion to set up in a position … treatment earlier than this is easier;

also along this same line of wisdom … symptoms occur thirty-six and a half hours after the real cause … not the apparent cause … Alan did a lot of work on this with a neurophysiologist, and I have found it invaluable when searching for cause rather than blaming bacteria for infections (for example) or a fall as the cause of an injury … again, what is behind the scenes, what is hidden from our bias is the Foundation of Osteopathic Thinking … "Find the Cause, where is the Fulcrum, and interface with Laws not framed by human hands" … this is the map for our journey in Biodynamics and is the cause for our thinking and principles.

Alan Becker was a Great Osteopath. He brought his brother Rollin to meet Will … Alan was a joyful inquiring soul … he was kind and radiant … in the last years of his life, he shared a great deal with me. He liked the Biodynamic work; I sent him tapes with questions, he answered, and we talked in ease … may he rest in the arms of his Beloved … gratefully, we remember him with love.

AUTOMATIC SHIFTING REVIEW

A. The Neutral is vital

B. Automatic Shifting Fluid Body
   1. Synchronization with Primary Respiration
   2. Tempo of the observer
   3. Precision is infinite, as is the potential in the moment
   4. Void may not be necessary

C. Therapeutic forces vs. effects of treatment
   1. Stay with therapeutic agencies
   2. Avoid:
      a. Compensatory fluid motions
      b. Barriers
      c. Therapeutic effects:
         1. Last longer than therapeutic input
         2. Tissue motion is always an effect
      d. Augmentation; we augment through synchronization
   3. Observe the specific and the global

D. The Access
   1. 2–3 cpm
   2. Void
   3. Wait—sense of fluid sea
   4. Minnow appears
   5. May occur without void

E. End point
   1. Pattern ends at a specific site
      a. Notation for next visit
      b. Forces recede to midline like a CV4

c. Stillpoint or pause
    1. If pause, may go to Long-Tide then convert to 2–3 cpm
d. Chart pattern of work done by Automatic Shifting

F. Rebalancing at End of Treatment. We are never a "perfect" act of conscience

$E=MC^2$

Energy Mass and the Speed of Light

Inertia And Momentum

A Lesion field has Energy in it ... we call it Inertia ... that Energy is involuting, it is not static.

A Lesion Field has motion in it ... we call it Momentum, or the Thread connected to the Health ... that Energy is evolving, it is not static.

At every second we are either going one way or the other, but nothing stays static in any form or function.

The E of the energy in the Lesion Field is the potential energy that, if released, will provide momentum toward Wholeness and healing.

The E equals the Mass of the Lesion Field times the speed of light: $E=MC^2$

If the Potential Energy in the Inertia is equal to the Mass of the lesion times the speed of light (C^2) ... that's a lot of Energy.

In order to get all the potential energy in the equation released, the equation must move as a unit of Function ... it must be Neutral, not adding conditions to the equation ... then it Transmutes ... as it does, the equation changes to ... $EM=C^2$ ... so that the Inertial Energy and the Mass are one ... then, using the Stillpoint, the C^2 (the Potency) moves with the mass as one ... and we have $EM=C^2$ as a Wholeness, not as an equation.

Seeing Mass and Energy and Light as different only defines a partitioned system; Einstein kept moving the equation from right to left ... I do not understand him, but I see Beauty here in this Wholeness.

I believe we are seeing Relativity in action and only miss its activity when we insist on seeing Energy or Mass or the Potency as different places rather than as a Singularity in One Place ...

Dr. Wales often spoke of Inertia and Momentum in relationship to Lesions. She was a wonderful teacher ... she was precise and patient ... her hands reflected Wholeness into the Lesion, and as it Remembered the Light, it Died into the Health and its Wholeness ... she was a Mother to many ... who love her dearly ... Eternally Grateful are we.

PHASE THREE OVERVIEW

There is a Thread that connects all motion to the Health.

Phase One was about the Motion Present in the tissue and fluid. In Phase Two, we studied the Motions of the Fluid Body and the Indwelling Therapeutic Process called Automatic Shifting.

What causes Automatic Shifting? Why is it so precise in its timing and diagnostics? Dr. Still and Dr. Sutherland identified the Source in a variety of ways ... but once we added the understandings of Dr. Blechschmidt, what may have been seen by many as Philosophy or Spirituality became a true Science—which it already was, but many did not hear and see the truth in Osteopathy.

"The Health" is in everyone, an indwelling, complete perfection that is as incarnate as your fingers. The Intelligence of the Mechanism, which is behind the cause of creation, is in and through the Health, as stated by all three of the above teachers.

We are cared for twenty-four hours a day. If we become Neutral, the Health transmits a Therapeutic Force that is intimately aware of our Wholeness and our Lesion Fields ... Treatment is prioritized in a Wholistic Perspective, not in a symptomatic or psychological manner.

The goal of healing is to return to a partnership and friendship with the Health, which contains all of what is truly oneself.

Therapeutic forces are already intimate within the Lesion Field. They are there from the moment the insult occurs. These forces are waiting for the doorway to open ...

They will not force anyone to be healed ... they wait for neutral or direct synchronization before a healing process can begin.

In Phase Three, we look into the Lesion Field for the presence of the Long-Tide as an indwelling therapeutic force, waiting.

The Long-Tide has a rate of one hundred seconds per cycle ... we call it the Soft Potency because it heals with a Feminine Sweetness. It juxtaposes the Lesion but does not penetrate it ... rather the Lesion melts into it.

To study this Indwelling Therapeutic Force we will further explore the central nervous system ... especially the wholeness in the meninges (membranous coverings) of the brain and cerebellum ...

In Phase Three, we will also begin our Study of the Immune System and its requirements for healing ... this will lead us to the next level of Stillness called the Dynamic Stillness ... which will be our focus in Phase Four.

THE POTENCY

The word "potency" was chosen by Dr. Sutherland because it brings to mind a feeling of great power. The language Sutherland developed began in the late 1930s. As he grew in his work, the word implied something bigger and bigger until it carried the implication of a Divine Power that was unerring and capable of the miraculous.

If you hear the word "potency," you can only hope that the speaker or writer clarifies the context in which it is being used. The word became a popular term, but the meaning of it was almost frayed to death by overuse ... sometimes people spoke with pride that they "worked with the potency." In the Biodynamic Model, we have kept the word but clarify each type as either Potency with a capital *P* or potency with a small *p*.

Potency with a big *P* is used to distinguish the Creative Power of the Potency from its effects, denoted by our little *p* potency, which is the fluid in the fluid, or reciprocal tension potency.

There is only One Potency and several little potencies. The little potencies are powerful in their own right and have the capability to transmute, depending upon the Landscape (rate-related).

Little potencies can be controlled (if skill is refined enough) by the Osteopath. Big *P* cannot be directed by human intention. This distinction is very important.

In Phase Two, we began to separate the tissue, the fluid, and the fluid in the fluid (potency).

Why bother? Are they not one function?

Yes, they are one function, even one substance, but only when the system is nearly perfect. When we lesion, this one Substance fractures into layers of independent compensation (for safety).

These layers have rates of breathing and landings called tissue, fluid, and potency, because of their "nature." When lesioned, one acts like Tissue, one acts like Fluid, and one acts like an electromagnetic force (little potency), or "fluid in the fluid."

The Potency cannot lesion, and neither can the Health. The division into three functions is relative to the lesion field as a whole, not to the Health itself.

In Phase Two, we also studied the "fluid in the fluid" (fluctuations).

The Longitudinal and Lateral fluctuations do not behave like fluid but rather pass through the fluid like a shadow. This potency is only seen in this form at two to three cycles per minute. The fragmentation of the potency when broken (disruptions in the axial fluctuations) requires a CV4 or EV4 to create a Neutral, through which the Indwelling Therapeutic Forces can transmute the Fluid Body and its geometric flow.

This understanding from Sutherland is a deep and profound truth that will serve to help the Tide do its great work.

We come to understand that potency needs a Neutral to be able to heal us.

This idea is not new... Hoover taught Sutherland about Neutral in relationship to Thoracic Respiration. Later Sutherland understood its relationship with Primary Respiration.

The capacity for Neutral conditions the capacity for transmutation.

Phase Two was therefore arranged to help you understand the potency and Neutral at a distinct level of compensation (2–3 cpm). If a Neutral is accomplished, the Potency can repair the potency and the Fluid Drive can express an Indwelling Capacity to Heal, i.e., Automatic Shifting.

There is a form that potency creates; we call this Zone B.

There are similar activities that should not be confused with this potency: auric field, life force, vital energy, and chi. These energies are real and are connected with other systems within the Whole.

Dr. Fulford, Dr. Stone (Polarity Therapy), Chinese Acupuncture, and Homeopathy all have made great contributions to healing. These other energies circulate in different pathways and are not synonymous with the Osteopathic term "potency." They function under different Laws and are ordered by different Principles.

Interestingly, when Still talked about Life as a force, he said, "Life is a slow vivifying force sent forth from Deity." ... to me this reflects a POTENCY of another dimension.

Having seen this first level of Fluid Body activity in Phase Two, we now move onward to Phase Three and a different kind of Potency: the "Soft Potency" or Long-Tide. This Potency moves slowly and cannot be directed unless one is perfectly synchronized with its tempo (moves like the tempo of the sun in the sky, one hundred seconds per cycle, fifty seconds each phase). The tone and texture of this Potency is cloud-like, graceful, beautiful, and sweet. It heals by juxtaposition and waits until the lesion field senses its presence. For this reason, we call it feminine, as opposed to the little *p* potency at two to three cycles per minute, which is vectorial and heals by penetration of the lesion field, and which has more male characteristics (Jungian context). When the Long-Tide expresses form, we call it Zone D, The Sea Around Us.

Zone D extends from the Central Stillness inside you to the circumferential horizon. In this ocean are many wonderful activities that Phase Three begins the exploration of.

Now we have created a language for the Biodynamic Model: Zone

A, Zone B, and Zone D. But what about Zone C?

Zone C is our relationship with the Service of Helping Others, with Serving the Divine. It is a truly heartfelt wish to Serve. It is what Rollin Becker called the "spiritual fulcrum."

The Fluid body has many levels of activity that occur concurrently. The Long-Tide and the 2–3 cpm coexist until a certain healing is accomplished in the whole.

It is a polyrhythmic system that also has levels of activity with no rates ... such as the Dynamic Stillness, The Health, and Wholeness. Where there is no rate, the Potency with a capital *P* is the power that generates a therapeutic process and vitalizes function.

The Potency with a capital *P* cannot be effective if the clinician has any desire to control the outcome of the treatment.

It is discernment, not a theoretical understanding, that distinguishes this profession. Words express the Art of Osteopathy; the Science follows.

Sutherland carried his Art through into a language and a model for Primary Respiration. He was still searching until just before his death.

When asked what he thought moves the fluids, he said, "I don't know." (This was a direct conversation between Will and Anne Wales in 1953, reported to me by Anne.)

After sixty years, Sutherland was still ready to be a beginner.

The first edition of *Osteopathy in the Cranial Field* is his true work. If you have not read it, then you have not seen the whole story. Magoun edited out a great deal trying to make the work more scientific. In my opinion, he failed to accomplish popularizing the work as he had hoped to.

THE SOFT POTENCY AND THE FLUID BODY

The world around us is precious ... yet ... we tend not to notice the Presence of the Long-Tide ... we have lost our background music ... the sound we were born to hear is all but drowned in a sea of inner and outer "noises."

A car swishes by ... after it passes ... the air is still ... filled by a sweet, sweet movement that embraces the Heart so purely ... the breath ends ... Nourished beyond words ... Wholeness rises up ... fragrant to the point of grief ... slowly recalled.

It is not too often that one meets something so Beautiful that it overshadows one's compensatory purpose ... such is the Long-Tide ... motion with Presence, patience, power, and intention ... No, it is not the Breath of Life ... but who sends this messenger?

As we work with the Long-Tide, it will most likely convince you that you are loved and that the Health is "nearby." ... It will make you feel its absence with a Grief that has been buried in sound and fear forever ... it is not a biological force ... it Lives and has a Mind that is Singular in its desire to restore the Blueprint of Life ... the Image of the Health in you ... never by force ... it sits next to the Lesion and waits ... waits ... as long as necessary.

It is known by Instinct, not knowledge ... it is part of the history of the human race from aboriginal to prophet ... it is known by many names ... it is a wind that carries a story, a story written in our Hearts ... sacred beyond Secret ... whose absence is felt as a need for Help in the souls of those who wish to remember.

It is a Fluid in the Fluid of the Sea Around US ... Zone D.

It passes through and vivifies Zone B.

It moves from the Central Stillness to the periphery ... it comes from the Periphery to the Central Stillness from many directions ... it is soft like a cloud ... patient in an eternal sense of time ... warm, hot, molding the Whole without parts ...

The purpose is to restore the Wholeness of the Fluid Body, from a condition of displacement from Zone A or internal lesioning from any cause.

RESUSCITATION: EV4, SOFT POTENCY

Practical

Center Your Hands Behind the Diaphragm

The Purpose Is to Sense the Whole of Zone B as One Drop

This Is Very Important in the Internal Dynamics of the Fluid Body.

Find a Place to Work From That Is Easy for You ...

Sense the whole of Zone B without Zone A.

Wait for your mind to be neutral so that Zone B is easily "seen."

During the inhalation phase of Primary Respiration, there are two motions from the Central Stillness ...

One is two to three cycles per minute and is vectorial.

One is very slow and soft like a cloud ... This is the "soft potency."

Note the soft potency and how far from the center to the periphery it moves ... Usually it is a few inches ... Normal is a motion from the center to well outside the skin where it creates a form ... The boundary of Zone B ... This is rare.

To Treat:

Synchronize with the tempo of the soft potency.

Wait.

Augmentation should occur, with no further intention.

The soft potency transmutes ...

Moldable liquid appears (sometimes).

Zone B merges with Zone D ...

Stillness lasts a while or more.

Zone B ... returns as breathing on the Long-Tide ... 100 seconds per cycle.

There are many variations.

MEDITATION: THE SEA AROUND US AND THROUGH US

Dr. Sutherland describes the sea around us and through us ... As if we were transparent.

We call this aspect of Primary Respiration Zone D. It is Breathing. From the horizon to the Central Stillness inside you, there is an Ocean filling the space ... one quality is the ebb and flow of its presence.

One method of clarifying this is to Sense your Breathing (thoracic), the Spiritual Stillness in the Room, and the Ocean Breathing. All three of these will be seen at the same time ...

If you get too technical, the awareness cannot become Whole ... the awareness wants to become Whole, so if you are Neutral to the task it will happen easily and deeply as follows ...

Let your mind see one of the three phenomena ... let it pick one for itself ... then watch the mind automatically shift from one phenomenon to another in what appears to be a random sequence ... let it roam from one phenomenon to the other ... it will collect toward the Wholeness of Thoracic Respiration, the Spiritual Stillness, and the Motion of the Long-Tide coming through you ... they can, and often do, blend and reveal a higher aspect of the Sea Around Us ...

Let it work ... watch ... There is an indwelling motion toward Normal ... a constant and instinctual need in us to be Whole ... with the Health ...

THE MENINGES AND THE LONG-TIDE

We will continue our studies of the development of the Central Nervous System that we began in Phase One. We will engage the indwelling therapeutic presence of the Long-Tide in the Lesion Field as our primary Principle of Treatment.

As you recall, embryological movements that create the shape and form of the Embryo are exact and momentary. The whole is changing as a Singularity, not in pieces as one might tend to think.

After reviewing Sutherland's recording about the Lamina Terminalis as the fulcrum for evolutionary motions of the central nervous system, we discovered that he was decades ahead of contemporary Embryology in his understanding of many things.

We discussed the Fluid as a protoplasmic field (not as water ... we saw how Space opens in the Fluid Body and Function moves into that Space easily without force ... the order being from an Intelligence much more refined than the central nervous system. Sutherland called this Mind "the Breath of Life," "the Tide," and the "Mechanism." All these terms reflect unerring, perfect Potency of a Supreme Intelligence.

We discussed the creation of the Cerebral Cortex ... the neurons being at first clustered around the third ventricle ... the Fluid Space around the third ventricle was quite wide ...

At a predetermined moment, the Fluid Field internally took on the form of a tree (arborization) ... this form was empty space ... as the Space opened, the cells moved outward from the third ventricle ... they went into the Space and Form created Biodynamically by the Intelligence of the Tide.

The motion of cells filling the form was without resistance; the cells moved in the Direction of Ease and finally came to rest as the

Tissue of the Cerebral Cortex ...

This arborization is essential to Growth and Healing ... it requires a stress-free fluid (Neutral).

In children, once this Space opens there are two million synapses per second that appear as the ultimate potential is expressed ... the synapses appear and disappear until the balance point is reached in the child's brain ... How and why is this done? One can only be awed by the potential.

In Phase One we also observed the Cranial Bones as a unit of function. We proposed that the sutures open as a unit and create the Space for the bones to breathe into, noting that the bones could transmute from the beginning of the Inhalation Phase to the end ... This, of course, is the same Principle as in the Arborization of the Cortex ... Space opens in a shape, and function moves into the form of the shape. The Cause is in the Potency of Transmutative fire of Primary Respiration.

The Meninges are the covering upon the Brain. The word comes from the Greek. Aristotle referred to the Meninges as the Membranes of the Brain ... a term Sutherland picked up when he coined the term "Balanced Membranous Tension" (BMT) as a method of treatment for the cranial bones.

Sutherland also used the term "Reciprocal Tension Membrane" (RTM) to describe the basis of meningeal activity associated with the Brain as a force united within the movement of Primary Respiration.

Our discussion today is in his honor and is not an effort to outthink Sutherland, but rather to further enjoy the unveiling of his work and discoveries.

The story begins, as usual, with the Protoplasm's neutrality ... just being ... not waiting just Neutral ... empty of self-intention, but with the potential to become anything that Creation designs, as an incarnate reality. This is called the embryonic plate, a misnomer for sure!

The textbooks say that Protoplasm trilaminates into Ectoderm,

Mesoderm, and Endoderm, which it does. But the formula is so rigid that one can miss the biological process and think anatomically about a dance that is a Living and Dying process ... the kaleidoscopic dance continues, but the dancers die and new dancers appear, moment to moment.

Imagine a treatment that never stops!

The Meninges are sacs, bags that are shaped by the Tide and provide very different functions. They all arise from the Mesoderm and have unique cellular components, making each sac functionally different.

The Leptomeninges are finer and smaller than the other membranes. They embrace the Cortex and have a layer of cerebrospinal fluid between them ... the pia mater is the most intimate and the arachnoid mater the most peripheral. Both the pia and the arachnoid completely embrace the Brain in a sac-like manner, with cerebrospinal fluid between them in a "subarachnoid space."

Lepto: Greek, fine, thin, delicate

Pia mater: Latin, "tender mother"

Arachnoid mater: Greek, "spider's web"

Microscopically, the words are accurate.

Peripheral to the arachnoid is another "sac" ... the dura mater. This dura mater is mislabeled by anatomists as the "tough mother," which it is not ... embalmed or dry specimens that Sutherland observed give a grave picture compared to the living dura mater, which is as fine as wet Kleenex ... this observation was made many times by Stefan Hagopian, D.O., in the dissections he has done over the past twenty-five years ... a point to remember!

The Dural sac has been conceptually placed aside by the three sickles of the reciprocal tension membrane. In basic courses, there still persists an insistence on seeing the Dura as three sickles acting as ligaments, moving and ordering the bones in their passive response to the motion of the cranial base. The reciprocal tension membrane refers to a membranous tension that is constant and shifts position around the junction of the falx and the tent. This means that the membrane does not transmute, nor do the bones breathe as a primary response to the Tide. This is not true—they do.

In 1954, Sutherland clearly said he was not sure what was creating the Fluid motions (see Anne Wales letter, in Biodynamics of Osteopathy Phase Two), thus abandoning the above model of the reciprocal tension membrane.

The sac of the dura mater is remarkably diverse. It travels peripherally along all nerves, and so it does not end in anatomy but in histology. The slides speak for themselves.

Above the Dural sac is a space ... the Epidural Space ... we are told that it is not present in adults, but functionally it is. The periosteal sac has a different makeup, a different nerve and blood supply. In newborns, we have consistently found an epidural space, and embryology confirms this to be the true shape of the developmental fields. There are fontanelles in the newborn skull not seen in the dura mater, which inclines one to see these sacs as different "places of functional specificity" ...

Anatomists prefer to make the internal periosteum and the dura mater one layer ... they are not.

In the next layer of the developing Ectomeninx of the Periosteal sac, the bones are expressed in between layers of outer and inner periostea. The periosteum begins as one layer ... as growth occurs, the bony elements appear within this one layer, creating two layers ... An infant's head easily demonstrates the single layer of tissue at the fontanelles ... the bones grow inside a single sac that becomes partitioned, anatomically but not functionally ... the sac with all the bones lesions as a unit of function; interosseous lesions are less common than one might think ... Dr. Wales often stressed the fact that balanced membranous tension was not about the bones being moved but rather their embracing of membrane (periosteum) ... That's why it is called balanced membranous tension … she said it was the most difficult thing for people to adjust to … not the bone, but the membrane is where the balance point is pursued.

The caput succedaneum in newborns is outside the periosteal sac and manifests as edema in the scalp and superficial layer, while a cephalohematoma is in the periosteal sac and thus does not cross the immature suture lines (single layer).

Embryology makes diagnosis easy … Anatomy makes it confusing.

Inside all this is a therapeutic force … waiting.

THE MENINGEAL SACS

Practical

We will evaluate the cranium by observing the functioning of the tissues relative to their involuntary motions (motion present) … this includes the Periosteal sac, the sac of the dura mater, and the intrinsic motions of the brain.

This will create a foundation for diagnostics that will be refined in time.

Anytime you evaluate the head for injury, this will serve as a good starting point.

Synchronize with the Health.

The sacs begin on the outside, not the inside, so looking inside for information is not helpful … Sense the Outer Layers … the Skin, the Muscular, and the Periosteal; all kinds of clinical issues can be clarified by knowing these layers … especially in head trauma … and newborns.

Sense for the periosteal sac, without any sense of bony tissue (hardness) … Sense the inner and outer periosteal tissues as one layer.

What is the normal tone of this tissue?

How does or does not the sac move during Inhalation? How much Inertia is present? Where is the fulcrum for the Inertia?

Where is the fulcrum for the normal motion in the anterior, middle, or posterior cranium?

During the Inhalation Phase, how does the sac change from the first third, to the middle third, to the last third of Inhalation … does it transmute or not?

***Keep your attention divided between the Health and the Tissue activity ... too much focus can make it a "long day." ... Ninety percent on the Health ... not the task at hand!

What happens to the texture as the Inhalation Phase processes? Does it resist? Does it wait? Does it join in easily and dance in the window of fire (inhalation)? Does it have a personality?

If you try to engage the tissues (balanced membranous tension) ... direction of ease, how little force brings the tissue to the Balance point? ... do not treat, just predict ...

Wait for the patient to rebalance ... check from the feet.

THE DURA MATER

The Dura Mater Is Not as Tough as You Might Imagine from Its Name

This Meningeal sac is found using the difference in temperature from the Periosteal sac ... just stay with the Health and notice the temperature of the Periosteal sac and sense for a warmer sac ... do not use tissue form or texture to find it, just temperature, please ... overzealousness will cloud the senses.

Check for its response to inhalation ... does it transmute as easily as the periosteum?

Does it transmute at the beginning, middle, or end of the inhalation phase?

What is its persona ... does it dance like a curtain in the wind as the periosteum does, or is it more stern?

What moves it?

If you tried balanced membranous tension on this tissue, the patient would react with meningeal irritability ... as many have discovered, this tissue is not agreeable to being pulled on ... meningeal irritability is a seriously sickening experience ... with headache, nausea, photophobia, and disequilibrium ...

Where is the fulcrum to which it spatially orients itself?

Rebalance from the feet.

Check the Brain ... Not the leptomeninges, as they are intimate to the central nervous system and rarely need isolated attention ... Note central nervous system motion as we did in Phase One ... then check for rebalancing again.

TREATMENT

First, which area needs help the most?

Are all the sacs synchronized or is one lagging behind? What sac has the most motion?

Make your diagnosis ... then we will find the presence of the Long-Tide in the Lesion Field, step into its motion, synchronize, and the treatment will express itself ... what if you make the "wrong" choice? No worries, the Long-Tide will move to the correct tissue and you will be learning from its wisdom.

Notice the style of the therapeutics related to the Long-Tide and how different it is from balanced membranous tension or Automatic Shifting at two to three cycles per minute.

Check the Wholeness of the Fluid Body and rebalance.

LANGUAGE, PHASE THREE

Language in Osteopathy can be a "rocky road." Terminology is often modified from teacher to teacher without clarification.

Sutherland was a journalist ... he carefully chose his words, many of which he probably took from Dr. Still.

The purpose of language, for an Osteopath, is not the theoretical usage of words ... for the words must describe what one has observed while treating.

This profession is an oral tradition and an empirical science, based upon observations of Natural and Divine Laws that are "not framed by human hands."

Potency: This word has multiple references with several meanings. The multiplicity comes from having used the word earlier in this work and then needing it in later years to describe a new form of power. "Potency" means "innate power" in the case of Primary Respiration. It means the power that organizes a therapeutic process. In Biodynamics, I have attempted to solve the confusion in several ways ...

First, we use the word potency generically for any power related to the Fluid in The Fluid ... and the Potency with a big *P* to mean the Absolute Overshadowing Power of the Intention of the Breath of Life.

Second, the potency with a little *p* is controllable by the will of the operator; that is, the potency can be managed or directed ... this, of course, is not true for Potency with a capital *P*, which cannot be managed by the will of the operator.

Third, the potency I usually refer to is a Fluid in the Fluid, even though sometimes the word "fluid" is meant in a broader sense to include this. The Fluid in the Fluid is an electromagnetic force ... In the first edition of *Osteopathy in the Cranial Field*, Sutherland calls it "current." ... Direct current is the Longitudinal Fluctuation, and indirect current is the Lateral Fluctuation.

These comments refer to the behavior of potency at two to three cycles per minute. These references are to potency with a small *p*. Additionally, we have found that the potency of the Long-Tide (100 seconds per cycle) can be managed, and, though more powerful than the potency at 2–3 cpm, it is still a small *p* potency.

The capital *P* potency refers to the Cause of Primary Respiration, the Breath of Life, and the Divine Love ... the Absolute Power of Creation ... the power to perform the Miraculous. Each kind of potency has a different sensation ... discernment of the differences is the hallmark of skill and communication.

The tide and the Tide, the stillness and the Stillness, the stillpoint and the Stillpoint—all have similarities to the above discussion.

Primary Respiration: The effects of the breathing of the Breath of Life.

The Breath of Life: It is not definable, but certainly one can say that it is the Anima ... the animating force of Creation, coming forth from Divine Love. The Wind that passes through everything as if it was Transparent, creating the Moment ... the Movement of Eternity into incarnation.

Dynamic Stillness: This is also called Third Level Stillness. It is the Substance that is molded by the Breath of Life to Create the Health in everything. It is Potency with a capital *P*. We first used this term in 1988, many years before the publication of Dr. Becker's work; the coincidence for me represents the fact that the world of Primary Respiration, if followed using Will Sutherland's method, is knowable and communicates Itself to us ... what we find is universal.

The Long-Tide: A breathing of cloud-like potency through us at a rate of 100 seconds per cycle. It is from the Sea of Zone D. Dr. Becker brought us to this rate, and much has been done in response to his bidding.

Zone D: Zone D is the space that a natural mind operates within ... it extends from your Central Stillness to the horizon ... it is an Aboriginal awareness of the Natural World and its internal communication ... children, elders, and mystics all live here at the base level of perception.

Zone C: The spiritual fulcrum around which one gathers oneself into Service ... it has spatial dynamics that can be from oneself or from the Tide Itself ... see the 1965 Sutherland Memorial Lecture, given by Rollin Becker, D.O.

Central Stillness: Not a Midline, nor it is usually understood; rather a Dynamic Stillness that is formless but can give rise to form. It is a doorway to the Sea Around Us.

Ignition: This goes back to Dr. Still and "The Engine of Life Fired by the Divine Spark" ... the ultimate Potency that vivifies life. It fires up the Fluid Body, gives it the drive and potency to do its work. It vivifies the immune function.

Transmutation: The change of something into a completely different state ... a change of essential nature or species.

Pause: A place of resynchronization ... with the true Midline parts that have been transmuted.

Stillpoint: A place of Potency and transmutation.

SEGMENTATION OF THE DURA MATER

The concept of three sickles in the Dural sac needs revision.

The research to support the questions arising when one takes a Biodynamic View of Primary Respiration has taken thirty years ...

Concerning the dura mater, we set out to research all of what was proposed in the Basic texts and courses, using fresh dissections. As we saw, the sacs are unique in form and function.

The dura mater has many folds. One of the first outcomes of rereading anatomy and embryology and doing dissections was the realization that there are two tents ... this was so obvious that I wondered, how could this truth have been overlooked? There are many reasons ... but now we are able to see clearly that there is a sac around the cerebrum and one around the cerebellum; these two sacs interface and eventually juxtapose and share fibers but retain their individual function.

In children, the two layers (where the two sacs are proximate) grow at different rates, meaning that the tent cannot be evaluated and/or treated as a single tissue. This changes the view of supra occiput and interparietal occiput in that they embrace two different zones of growth tempo.

Additionally, children have a functional epidural space, which means the bones do not have poles of attachment connecting the dura and the periosteum ...

We need to trust what we feel, even if the book does not mention it ... that is how we got to this place.

The Art of Osteopathy has created the Science from empirical observation, not the other way around. This is our Tradition.

The dura mater has at least eighteen layers in all (so far), which, as you will see, are not truly duplications but separate layers that have moved from being separate functions to being together as a single two-layered function. The falx, for example, is formed from two venous channels that slowly merge as the meninges journey toward their final form/position.

Anyone under the age of twenty-eight is officially not finished with dural growth ... a child treated as an adult is limited by anatomical misunderstandings, but if an adult is treated as a child, the functional interfaces will be respected and the clinical outcomes much better.

Anatomy does not exist in the manner in which we see it ... it is rather as Still saw it (see *Philosophy of Osteopathy*, chapter one ... What is anatomy?)

Today we will observe the layers of the dura mater and the space from which they are formed ... the space in between layers. This space contains the matrix that expresses the form.

The form does not create the space in between layers.

THE SEGMENTATION OF THE DURA

The Space That Creates Its Folds

The Long-Tide … Waiting

THE ANTERIOR DURAL GIRDLE

The story of the Anterior Dural Girdle is fascinating.

I want to stress that the Girdle is a Fluid Field, not a band of tissue ... the Field acts as a unit of Fluid (protoplasm and its progeny) ... and spans the area from the bregma to the xyphoid, and all functions therein. This will be clear as you treat.

In later Phases, we will give more consideration to its role in Osteopathic Thinking, but please do not let it become Anatomy to be manipulated, as this tendency is a great temptation and disruptive to the Soul of Wholeness ... it is not a thing, but rather a Greatness that defies our mental capacities ... our task is to cooperate and communicate with the "Laws not framed by human hands" (A. T. Still) ... Those laws are before us now.

THE BIRD AND THE IMMUNE RESPONSE

There are many "forms" in the Cranium ... the Sphenoid and the Neural Tube certainly look like Birds, and perhaps this symbolism means something.

In "The Tour of the Minnow," Sutherland describes the bird-like flight of the Neural Tube (the ventricles, the brain stem, and the spinal cord). This is our first brain, and the consciousness is interactive and severely acute. It is millions of years old in its wisdom.

The Bird, as we view it in today's work, is about the core consciousness of the Immune System ... the Immune System, as you know, can sense self and non-self entities and make a clear response ... many patients do not make a clear discernment and response, and so autoimmune disease develops ... often disabling ... clarity depends upon a "lack of noise" in the system as a whole. Rest/neutral are real needs.

The Immune System is formed from Self, which precedes the division of "self/non-self" partitions. Any book that reviews the embryological development of the Immune system will discuss this transition from Self (Health) to a self/non-self system. The standard medical texts on disease are not worth the time; a text on the Development of the Immune system is invaluable ... try *The Neuro-Immune-Endocrine Connection* by Carl Cotman et al., published by Raven Press ... Also look for texts written on the research of the beginnings of the Immune System and of Consciousness ... remember, *perception* is an immune function.

The Core Consciousness of the Immune System is vigilant! It watches and reacts to millions of pieces of data ... it is therefore in need of Rest ... Neutral ... and rarely gets the "time" because WE DO

NOT REST. So on it goes day after day being overloaded by our minds and intentions ... To do good work, the Immune System needs quiet ... that is, a low level of synaptic noise in the central nervous system ... THIS COMES ONLY WITH REST ... NOT RECREATIONAL PLEASURES ... How can we create the environment for the recovery ... how can we get the Bird into a Neutral? What are the consequences of such compared with CV4/EV4?

In 1982, I began working on this question. A review of Sutherland's writing yielded only one comment on the CV3 ... his approach was from the posterior parietal region and he said that he used it for hypertension ... the brief comment was all I could find. After our discovery of the Anterior Dural Girdle, I decided to try to use the tissue around the girdle to bring the third ventricle down to a Stillpoint, similar to CV4 ... but Something kept saying STOP! ... As I narrowed the transverse diameter of the girdle, I could feel a lateral fluctuation coming to meet my forces ... it said no, over and over ... using a variety of clever moves, it still turned me away ... I realized the third ventricle was V3 and not V4 and that the "centers" here were very highly refined ... so one day, after months of frayed efforts, I knocked on the door rather than trying to gain entrance ... I knocked quietly ... waited ... and from inside came a "flutter" ... strange? ... Again, I knocked ... again, a "flutter." ... well? I was in the dark, period. Time passed. I reflected upon "what's missing" in this event. What was the flutter?

I was being too conceptual and technique oriented ... what I needed was a sense of reverence and respect for the Mystery behind the whole Mechanism ... I knocked again, but this time I went to the Stillness that precedes all function arising from the area of the third ventricle ... a still, egg-shaped space larger than the third ventricle and at a level where no anatomy exists ... recognition of the Stillness Central to the arising of the third ventricle made <u>me</u> still inside ... it was quiet ... I waited ... holding my mind still, and disciplined upon the Stillness, listening for nothing ... a flutter came ... it was the Neural

Tube (the Bird) ... I inquired through Ignorance toward some help in understanding ... the Bird seemed to want to Rest upon Its Original fulcrum ... I realized it did not trust me ... Knowing the bird's level of responsibility, and the little anyone knows about the Brain and the Immune System, I set myself to unknowing ... then the Bird nestled down a little ... I felt like something great was in the air ... I got excited; the Bird looked at me the way a mother bear protects her child ... It was clear that the Bird was disgusted with my lack of being ... I waited and settled my Heart in Eternity ... and waited ... slowly and with a testing attitude the Bird went into a Resting posture ... aah, I thought, a Neutral ... the Bird unfolded as if awoken early ... I saw again my need for knowing ... and how that is not what Nature demands from us ... I rested in myself as best I could ... it was over ... no Rest came for the Bird, as I had awoken it early with my rationality.

Many returns and many apprehensions later, I found that the key to communication and trust was to let the attention be held by the fulcrum ... to stay with the Stillness and not waver ... then the Bird could trust me to hold the fulcrum while it Rested, Paused, and refreshed ... Using this orientation, the Bird came to Rest in treatment after treatment and the results were clinically evident.

When the Bird Rested, it became buoyant in a rich Dark Endless Stillness, beyond Zone D ... At first, I was scared ... the Stillness was an endless void like the Space between the Stars at night ... this New Stillness had a Magnitude; its emptiness was a call to something inconceivable ... Something distant ... a Presence ... coming.

The Bird Rested a long time, floating in the Vast Night of the Stillness ... I waited without inner commentary ... finally a Giant Shadow of a Bird rose up and spread its wings into Zone D, not A or B but D ... well, crazy or not, I held firm ... and waited ... even though I was challenged ... the tissue motion eventually returned and the vitality increased in the third ventricle and its relationships.

The new stillness was dynamic ... So I called it the Dynamic

Stillness, not knowing that Dr. Becker had done so himself (his books came out eight years later and someone told me about it) ... that alone lifted the story further into meaning.

As I used this understanding, clinical results came forward with unexpected refinement ... The first case was a child with a severe immunization reaction that left him, at five years old, with night fevers (104°) and frequent infections, and he was introverted all the time (autism) ... His outcome was 60 percent recovery after two sessions eight weeks apart. This after hundreds of specialist visits had not helped him in the least ... I have never seen a CV4 work this well ... It became clear after another five hundred cases that this CV3 ... the Bird ... was powerful. But the work presented a perceptual challenge that was mystical at the least ... the teaching has continued since 1991 ... and the feedback has been very positive ...

Why have I written SO much? Well, as it turns out, after I introduced this to the profession, people began to use force on the system and quote me as the source ... this is not accurate. Any force applied here to this area will produce side effects that can be serious! Such as emotional fragility, several months after the treatment, that is severe. I have had to treat several of these, and although I continue to caution people, they persist in using direct action ... that's why I am so zealous ... also ...

The Health has taught me Its wishes in regard to this area, and for me that is Law ...

In *A Manual of Cranial Technique* by the Lippincotts, on the first page, Sutherland clearly makes a case against direct action ...

These are three good reasons to walk quietly, especially in the arena of the Dynamic Stillness that cannot be accessed "directly." ... Learn to communicate rather than dictate ... communicate with a Greater Mind than ours in order to be safe and maximally effective ...

there continue to be books listing direct action techniques, with my name on the directions ... astounding ... even after several direct, one-on-one sessions with the authors, there still persists a need to "do things to the Brain."

... I believe we, as humans, are truly deaf to anything that requires us to be Neutral, to Listen, or to Treat Life as if It Knew ... may we all change.

Thank you ...

THE NEUROBIOLOGICAL BASIS OF FEVER

In *Surgical Neurology,* Issue 45, Amir Samii, M.D. (1996) writes:

> The mechanisms which are involved in the febrile response can be separated into three groups: endocrine and metabolic responses, autonomic responses, and behavioral responses. ...
> The immune challenge results in production of various proteins, called endogenous pyrogens (ENP), which are synthesized by phagocytic leukocytes. ...
> These large proteins are excluded by the blood-brain barrier ... .
> Specialized regions along the cerebral ventricular surface have no BBB. These areas are called circumventricular organs (CVO). The organum vasculosum of the lamina terminalis belongs to the CVO is thought to control the febrile response through projections to sites in the anterior hypothalamus and the brain stem .... ENPs can enter the organum vasculosum through fenestrated capillaries and may act on different cell types ... to induce the production of specific lipid metabolites called prostaglandins .... These prostaglandins seem to activate the organum vasculosum and/or the preoptic area which send axonal processes to other cell groups in the anterior hypothalamus and the brain stem and orchestrate the febrile response. ...
> The region around the organum vasculosum contains the highest levels of prostaglandin receptors in the entire brain ....

THE STORY WITHIN

In the center of the Bird's heart grows the divine spark, the common ground of all life. The Bird lives obediently by natural law, "by the rules." This is not perceived as a prison by the bird but rather the embrace of a wonderful dynamic stillness, which curiously disappears from consciousness when the spark is forgotten. The embrace of stillness is home for the heart of the bird. Absence of this stillness causes self-doubt, separation, loneliness, insanity. Consciousness of the dynamic stillness is a part of all creatures, all living forms—even the stones and stars.

Each one knows and feels known by the warmth of its own spark.

One tiny part of a star inside the heart is a fulcrum that automatically shifts rather than judges or compares. Once the Bird forgets the stillness, great frustration and desire enter it. It cannot remember how to get home, it cannot rest; it feels hopeless, lost, unembraced; and yet, rest could awaken the dreamer to remembering. But the Bird cannot rest. The Bird in its frenzy to find peace does not rest; it will not rest. Unresolve prevails!

The Bird flies through its Life uncentered, working very hard at not remembering the glide on the wind and its embrace. If only it could rest—but it has forgotten how. It does not remember. The mind and the heart never pause, and so it goes on and on in endless tense flight.

Each day the Bird sits for a while in its nest. It relaxes a little, but very little. Sometimes it closes its eyes and thinks it is resting "away from it all." But the heart remains instinctively uneasy; there is no deep peace, no embrace of the long reach, of the Breath and Light of the Divine Essence.

So it goes, on and on. The Bird tries harder and loses ground. It is grief-stricken and myopic. No memory of the spark remains. Life is dim, productive but empty. The missing remains unconscious and time passes.

Perhaps death is the only doorway to the light. Something must be resolved.

The Bird makes a large pile of sticks and logs, dry old wood piled high into the air. For days and nights it works, gathering from far and wide everything it can find and building a collection. The bird sighs deeply, looking at the pile; it is bewildered, almost shocked at the form before it. It breathes deeply, softly, slowly until it comes to a point of acceptance, balance, and surrender. The bird strikes a flint, and a spark flies into the pile. The fire ignites. The old wood burns intensely. The bird disappears. White ash glowing in the setting sun is all that remains in the quiet-laden air.

Night rises. One tiny spark remains aglow in the night's eye, one spark glowing, alone. At the last sign of life, the spark quivers. Again it quivers; the curtain of ashes moves to reveal a form emerging through the remains. Stillness solidifies. Day breaks, and at the first new breath of life, the Bird rises up again, held in the embrace of a wonderful Dynamic Stillness. The Bird glides into Memory upon the Wind of the Living ... and Remembers.

Like the heart chambers, the ventricles are the chambers of the spirit. The heart of the spirit. Like the heart of the soul residing in the heart, the divine implant of our perfection stills itself almost silently upon the center of the third ventricular chamber.

Here, with each inhalation of Primary Respiration, the matrix of life reignites, fired by divine warmth and a sense of the eternal.

CHILDREN'S OBSERVATIONS

Children seven to nine years old were asked to observe their mind and report what they saw with their imagination.

Imagination: to picture to oneself something not present to the original five senses. It is used here to acknowledge imagination as a creative act of the highest degree of insight.

As the children observed their inner world, this is what they reported:

1. It felt like a sea of many people that were fighting over me. (Joana, grade 3)
2. My imagination works with the whole body and looks like crawling on grass. (Jason, grade 4)
3. Mine looks like a brain, feels like a big circle in my head. (JoAnn, grade 2)
4. My imagination is like a blob. It changes shape, size, and color. If you could feel it, it would feel slippery and spongy. It sops up ideas and squeezes them into one idea. It fixes it up so that it is as good as can be and sends it to my mind. My mind sends it to my hand and I do it. (Alon, grade 4)
5. It felt like someone was in a boat. It felt like I was in a boat. (Daniel, grade 3)
6. My imagination changes by the minute. Now it's in my stomach. (Jacob, grade 2)
7. Opening and closing. (Ryan, grade 2)
8. My mind has many thoughts. Today her thought is a bird. Not just any bird though! (Erin, grade 4)
9. Blue fire, fierce fire. (Daniel, grade 4)

10. I can't go inside my mind without going side to side. It's so windy. I find out that the wind is wavy, and it has special mittens to pick up things. (Renee, grade 3)
11. If it is trapped it feels like it is going to die. (Amy, grade 4)
12. Who-hee-hee-hee-hee-hee. (Keith, grade 4)
13. It wants to be free. It doesn't want to be in an enclosed area. It likes to just be a nice summer breeze. (Jennifer, grade 4)
14. Freedom! (Nicholas, grade 4)
15. Very, very wavy. (Angela, grade 4)

Instinct is present throughout our lives; it knows. The skill we seek is innate.

FATHER DURA

Here is a quote from a transcribed tape recording of Dr. Sutherland speaking in Pacific Grove, California, in July 1954.

> The outer and inner walls of Father Dura concern venous circulation....
> I want you to notice the cross on the interior – the lateral sinus and up to the function of the sagittal. Now the ossification center of the occipital squama is located between the walls of Father Dura at the center of this cross....
> The ossification centers are within the outer and inner walls of Father Dura, so when we mold the occipital bone ...laterally ...
> I want you to visualize what is occurring within the inner wall of Father Dura.... molding contact up to the sagittal and include the inner wall ...
> The outer wall is merely the contact of convenience. See what occurs in front of that, within the inner walls of Father Dura. Fluid within both walls. Ossification centers within both walls.
> ...
> Instead of growing together by a segment of Mother Dura shooting up between, we have a growing together which includes Father Dura – its outer and inner walls. Otherwise, if not for this differentiation, with Mother Dura up between, we would get obstructions of the main venous walls of the skull.

Willam Garner Sutherland, D.O., "Father Dura," from a tape recording made in Pacific Grove, California, July 1954

LONG-TIDE REFERENCES BY ROLLIN BECKER, D.O.

Recommended reading: *Life in Motion* and *The Stillness of Life* by Rollin E. Becker, D.O. Here are a few brief quotes where he mentions the Long-Tide:

"It took a full minute and a half for this large tide to come in … modifying the tropism of every cell …" (1986, Life in Motion, page 113)

"I have a feeling the slow tide is at work many more times than I am aware of …" (1983, Life in Motion, page 125)

"When this tidal wave reaches its maximum filling state, there is a brief pause and it then begins to ebb out." (1983, Life in Motion, page 124)

"Unlike the fast tide … the slow tide seems to be an inherent entity in itself …" (1983, Life in Motion, Page 125)

"The reciprocal balance interchange … is augmented by, the fast and slow tides …" (1983, Life in Motion, Page 118)

"The vitality factors of the fast and slow tides are fundamental aspects of these health principles." (1983, Life in Motion, Page 120)

"This second tide permeates the entire body unit …" (1983, Life in Motion, Page 118)

"Both tides are present in health and also in trauma and/or disease." (1983, Life in Motion, Page 118)

"Both tides are innate, inherent, and involuntary, self-regulatory mechanisms …" (1983, Life in Motion, Page 118)

"… a gradual welling expansion of tide-like fingers of fluid …" (1979, Life in Motion, Pages 58 to 59)

"It is a more massive-feeling tide with a gradual welling expansion of the whole being …" (1979, The Stillness of life, Pages 226 to 227)

"… this large, tide-like motion. …" (The Stillness of Life, Pages 49 to 50)

OSTEOPATHY – TAKING ITS RIGHTFUL PLACE

An Address Delivered at Osteopathy 2000, the Third Annual British Osteopathic Congress
The Commonwealth Institute, London, Saturday, March 11, 1995
Irvin M. Korr, Ph.D., Professor Emeritus, Kirksville (1975) and Texas (1990)
Colleges of Osteopathic Medicine

Here is a brief quote from this address:

> ...there were two overlapping periods in this century. The first was from 1900 to mid-century when the predominant diseases were the acute infectious diseases and the victims were mainly infants, children and young adults. ...
> By 1950, 89% of live born infants were surviving ... to the 50th year of life. ...
> So what is the state of health of all these older people? Not very good.
> I characterized the first half of the century as 'the lower the morbidity, the lower the mortality.' Now, 'the lower the mortality, the greater the morbidity.' ...
> They are not the acute infectious diseases of the first half of the century but are chronic degenerative diseases. ...
> While our health care system is so absorbed in late-stage

irreversible disease, millions of infants, children and young people are already embarking on the same life paths that culminate in those same diseases. We simply have to move upstream ...

The holistic approach of Osteopathy is to modify all the factors in a person's life in a more favorable direction so as to disencumber that in-built health care system. ... This is the ultimate role of the osteopath.

OSTEOPATHIC MAGAZINE, 1925

Nature's Way to Better Health

Here is an article from the 1925 Osteopathic Magazine called "Moderation, Thoroughness, and Longevity".

> That "most distinguished man of this nation," Dr. Charles W. Eliot, at 90, stands at ease for one and a half hours listening to tributes of honor, then makes a brilliant and unprepared reply, declaring eating moderately, sleeping at least 7 hours with window open, exercising regularly in the open air, avoiding stimulants, enjoying all natural delights without excess, with serene spirit, then ten minutes devoted affectionately each day to good books—indeed, to one book of the first order like the English Bible or Shakespeare, will make a man mentally rich.
>
> Beware Quack Doctors
> Below Is a Timely and Pertinent Editorial Recently Printed in the *Chicago Evening American.*
> Before you let anybody, massage expert, osteopath, or chiropractor, manipulate your spinal column, make sure the man understands his business. Scientific manipulation of the backbone, freeing nerves from pressure, and scientific Osteopathy, generally, is of greatest value, often making medicines unnecessary and doing what medicines cannot do.
> But beware of the "overnight" graduate, who has failed at something and decides that he will make a living twisting backbones.
> He can twist too well. Recently a railroad conductor underwent two treatments including vigorous twisting of the neck. Within two days he was paralyzed on one side, could not write his name. He got over it, with the loss of three weeks' time. Make sure your scientist is a scientist, not a reformed blacksmith. There are thousands such practicing.
>
> Chicago Evening American, April 22, 1925

Nature's Tonics

In the 1925 Osteopathic Magazine, Vera Radel D.O. writes:

> Too little attention has been paid to the necessity of rest as a conserver of force, as a means of maintaining health and consequently happiness ... Hurry and worry are more fatal than disease. The true physician teaches men, women and children how to combine activity with rest, ...
>
> There would be fewer chronic invalids, fewer cases of melancholia and neurasthenia if people as a whole took more vacations and fewer hypothetical tonics. Real tonics are drawn from the vast storehouses of nature—from sunshine, pure air, exercise, healthful food and sleep.
>
> Ella Adelia Fletcher has expressed so beautifully the influence of nature upon our imagination, and says in her book The Philosophy of Rest, "Get away into the woods where the trees will talk to you, or down on the sands by the seashore where every incoming wave will whisper messages of the throbbing vitality of which you are a part. ...
>
> Every moment of this intimacy with yourself is fraught with deepest significance, ...

Osteopathic Magazine, 1925. In the public domain.

THE PAUSE AND THE LANGUAGE OF SILENCE

Recommended reading: *Freedom and Destiny* by Rollo May, Ph.D. Dr. May (1909–1994) was a clinical psychologist, known for his work in existential fields of psychology. Here are a few brief quotes where he mentions the "pause."

"It is in the pause that people learn to listen to silence."

"Pause is the prerequisite for wonder."

"The length of time of the pause is, in principle, irrelevant."

"The pause for milliseconds while one speaks is the locus of the speaker's freedom."

"The relation between creativity and the pause is as close as it is startling."

"... each of us experiences two aspects of selfhood which are never fully separated from each other. One of these aspects is the ego-self ... It judges the demands of reality, balances preconscious ideas, and sifts out unacceptable unconscious impulses so that the person can live with some unity ..."

"The other aspect is the psyche-self, which seeks to 'see life steadily and see it whole.' The psyche-self is concerned with the context of freedom. The 'heightened consciousness' of which we speak from time to time is a function of the psyche-self."

"... a higher level of consciousness, what was called 'oceanic' by Freud and Einstein. One experiences being absorbed into the universe and the universe being temporarily absorbed into one's self."

"In the holy void, the nothingness that we experience gives our deeper thoughts room to make themselves manifest, and the otherwise silent inner voice can be heard."

"The void is the dimension of eternity."

"... the spaces between words, the intervals, the pauses in life—these yield the touch of ecstasy ... may be experienced as a glimpse of God, assuming that God is conceived as the ground of being and meaning in the universe."

Rollo May, excerpts from *Freedom and Destiny* (Norton, 1981).

Go Outside and Listen as Far Away as You Can ...

What Transpires?

BIODYNAMICS OF OSTEOPATHY BOOK SERIES

This book is one of a series of twelve *Biodynamics of Osteopathy* books. It is recommended that you read the whole series in order, as each book builds on the understanding from prior books. It is also recommended that you seek experienced teachers and mentors to help you experience the full depth of the information given.

The full series is as follows:

Phase One is about involuntary motion, which is motion present in the whole and in the lesion. We learn to synchronize with the breathing of Primary Respiration before we approach any treatment. This synchronization is the key to working with stable rates and not irritating the system. The principle of synchronizing with a healthy aspect of the patient suffuses the whole teaching program. This synchronization shifts our awareness to a different level of receptivity, which allows us to see Primary Respiration rather than the lesion field, and this eventually leads us to an understanding of the intention of Primary Respiration.

Phase Two is about communication with the natural laws of healing that surround activity at 2 to 3 cycles per minute. We synchronize with the breathing of Primary Respiration and also add the skill of sensing the fulcrum, the Stillness through which the breathing creates form and function. It is a different kind of synchronization from that in Phase One, shifting our awareness more deeply. As this occurs, the treatment automatically expresses itself. The end point of treatment, when compared with Phase One, reveals several differences. We find this kind of synchronization works exclusively with the fluid body and the outcome of treatment is more complete than when working with tissue alone.

Phase Three is centered around the activities of the Long Tide (100 second cycle). We explore an indwelling therapeutic force already present in the lesion field. We learn that the dural system is not made-up of three sickles but rather a series of folds in a sac, arising during growth and development. We see the relationship between the upper and lower dural sacs, awakening us to the independence of two separate tentorium cerebelli. We discover that zone D, the horizon, and the Wire (along which the Long Tide moves during its intended therapeutic course) are all linked as natural laws pertaining to this level of Primary Respiration.

Phase Four focuses on the Midline, a place where the spatial relationships are expressed as a whole. It synchronizes and centers us in such a way that we become aware of Zone D and the Dynamic Stillness. The Third Level Stillness in Phase Four is different from the Stillness in the other Phases – we are centered by the Stillness at the center of creation. Our intention is replaced by the intention of the Tide which can facilitate our spiritual path.

Phase Five is about *the face*. As we approach the face, we use all of the principles that we have learned in Phase One, Two, Three, and Four. We work with automatic shifting and notice differences from how the face is viewed by older models within Osteopathy in the Cranial Field. As we synchronize with the therapeutic presence of the Long Tide we see what we can learn about the face from that landscape. We also work with Seams, Dynamic Stillness, and Ignition.

Phase Six is a continuation of our journey into the Wholeness that generates life and delivers therapeutic forces that transmute lesions once Neutral is expressed. It is a mixture of activities centered around the outside presence of Primary Respiration as something that is a non-biological force and that has a persona. We will also continue to explore seams and then move on to the extremities, first in the embryological terms and then as Sutherland taught them in his work called PowerPoints. Phase 6 is a time to build your understanding of the Tide and refine your skills.

Phase Seven highlights the Health. Dr. Still's famous comment "Find the Health; anyone can find disease," has plagued many minds over the last century. We come to the clear vision of several indwelling aspects of the Health: Love ... liquid light ... and a diamond matrix. A approach to the terminally ill and dying patient is addressed. In the somatic sensation of the Tide passing through the House Under the Sea, our awareness is transmuted by the Health. The lesion is seen as a precognitive act of the Health. Thoracic Respiration, Primary Respiration, and Ignition are as One. The landscape is vast ... and the principles of healing are even more substantial than we have previously experienced..

Phase Eight is a deeper exploration of seams, balanced rhythmic interchange, and the Flame of Intention as a therapeutic modality. Phase Eight is the culmination of our awareness of Wholeness, and ultimately brings us to the Divine Presence, Unconditional Love and Oneness. The living Tide dominates the awareness while forms move to the background. One feels the Breath of Creation in oneself as the Center of Wholeness. One feels the Unfoldment of oneself as one is Created. Our consciousness is a gift; we do not own it and if we try to control it we lose Wholeness.

Phase Nine is when we are able to fully evaluate and treat the

Central Nervous System and the Eye. We also address Fire and the therapeutic modality of the Shakedown. True action is moved from Love and makes our perception exist. This Love is self-emptying and by its nature allows us to Serve as part of the Perfect. Perception can be used to Serve something other than ourselves. We have attempted to enter this balance point between the Perfect and the Disease ... it is a point where the whole of everything is suspended by Love as it works to incarnate the Complete. In the balance point of everything is The Intention of the Tide following the movement of the distortion back to a True relationship with the Blueprint of Life.

Pediatrics One explores how children grow as a whole, not in parts as we sometimes believe. Children live in the Direction of Ease of motion present in their fluid metabolic fields, otherwise they get uncomfortable and require assistance. Does your treatment directly support the whole, or does it assume to support the whole? We realize children are not adults and cannot be treated as adults are. We approach the therapeutic modality of the "Meeting Place", prenatal and postnatal periods, the treatment of the pelvis during pregnancy, fetal malposition and labor.

Pediatrics Two is where we deepen in the perceptive awareness necessary to approach the treatment of children. We deepen in our appreciation of Wholeness, the three levels of Stillness and the "Meeting Place". We approach "Desert Neutral", where therapeutics pass into the neutral substance, and a mystery unfolds as the breath of Divine love cascades as a therapeutic force across a night desert landscape, filling and leaving behind no visible effects. We further address treatment of the pelvis and the uterus during pregnancy. We explore thoracic and Primary Respiration in children, and the Family Circle.

Pediatrics Three is where we continue to study the therapeutic

Flow of Attention. We deepen in Third Level Stillness and the Meeting Place. The Meeting Place is easily misinterpreted … our observer must be so still and neutral that the process can be seen as it happens. The central nervous system in the child can be finally approached for evaluation and treatment. We explore teething and also the "locked up head". We use the therapeutic modality of the Flame of Intention, and its connection to the Breath of Life. Everything is transparent to the Breath of Life.

ABOUT THE AUTHOR

James Jealous, D.O. (1943–2021), was an osteopathic physician, teacher, and writer. His life's work was founding and developing **Biodynamics of Osteopathy**, a unique methodology he established within the field of osteopathy, following the lineage of Dr. A.T. Still and Dr. W.G. Sutherland.

He was born in Saco, Maine, and since his father was an osteopathic physician, he was around osteopathy from an early age. He studied at Kirksville College of Osteopathic Medicine in Missouri (now the A.T. Still University of Health Sciences), graduating in 1970. He then set up practice in rural Maine as an osteopathic primary care physician.

Over time, Dr. Jealous saw parallels between the work of embryologist Dr. Erich Blechschmidt and that of osteopathic physician Dr. William Garner Sutherland. This inspiration led him to create his own body of work. In the early 1990s, he began teaching "A Biodynamic View of Osteopathy in the Cranial Field," which, as he developed his specific methodology, was refined to "Biodynamics of Osteopathy."

A deeply spiritual person, he felt most at home in the natural world and was an avid fisherman and hiker.

For more information, please visit:

https://BiodynamicsOfOsteopathy.com

There is a wind passing through . . .
it is the motion of creation,
the eternal motion of Divine love.